LOW POTASSIUM

DIET GUIDE FOR BEGINNERS

The nutritional guide on how to manage potassium levels for optimal renal health and benefit for people with chronic kidney disease with meal plan and a Food-list

Dr. RICKEY HARRY

Copyright © 2023 – Dr. Rickey harry

ISBN:
Printed in the United States of America

Disclaimer

This publication is designed to provide competent and reliable information regarding the subject covered. However, the views expressed in this publication are those of the author alone, and should not be taken as expert instruction or professional advice. The reader is responsible for his or her actions. The author hereby disclaims any responsibility or liability whatsoever that is incurred from the use or application of the contents of this publication by the purchaser of the reader. The purchaser or reader is hereby responsible for his or her actions.

All rights reserved. No part of this publication may be reproduced, distributed, or transmitted in any form or by any means, including photocopying, recording, or other electronic or mechanical methods, without the prior written permission of the publisher, except in the case of brief quotations embodied in critical reviews and certain other non-commercial uses permitted by copyright law. For permission requests, write to the publisher, addressed at the address below

TABLE OF CONTENTS

INTRODUCTION 7

    Reason for a low potassium diet 8

    Beneficiaries of a low potassium diet 10

OVERVIEW OF LOW POTASSIUM DIET 12

    Quantity of potassium needed 13

    Reasons for following a low-potassium diet ... 15

    Benefits of a low potassium diet 18

FOODS TO AVOID ON A LOW-POTASSIUM DIET .. 21

    High potassium fruits 21

    High potassium vegetables 23

    High-potassium protein sources 24

FOODS TO INCLUDE IN A LOW-POTASSIUM DIET . 27

    Low-Potassium Foods 27

    Low-potassium fruits: 27

    Other low-potassium foods: 29

    Procedure for leaching 30

A WEEK'S MEAL PLAN FOR A LOW-POTASSIUM DIET 32

Monday: 32

Tuesday: 34

Wednesday: 36

Thursday: 38

Friday 39

Saturday 41

Sunday 43

TIPS FOR PREPARING LOW-POTASSIUM MEALS 45

Cooking techniques to reduce potassium levels 45

Flavorings and seasonings to use 47

Tips for eating out on a low-potassium diet 49

Strategies for grocery shopping on a low-potassium diet 51

RECIPES FOR A LOW-POTASSIUM DIET 54

Grilled Chicken with Mango Salsa 54

Baked Salmon with Lemon and Dill 55

Quinoa Salad with Roasted Vegetables 56

Sweet Potato and Black Bean Chili 57

Grilled Vegetable Skewers 59

Lemon and Herb Baked Chicken 60

Quinoa Salad with Roasted Vegetables 62

Turkey and Vegetable Stir-Fry 63

Salmon and Asparagus Foil Packets 65

Low Potassium Turkey Chili 66

Low Potassium Vegetable Stir-Fry 68

Low Potassium Baked Salmon 70

Roasted Red Pepper and Feta Salad Recipe 71

Spicy Grilled Shrimp Skewers Recipe 72

Greek Yogurt Chicken Salad Recipe 74

Quinoa and Black Bean Salad Recipe 75

Baked Salmon with Lemon and Herbs Recipe
.... 76

Spicy Shrimp Stir-Fry Recipe 78

Quinoa Salad with Roasted Vegetables Recipe
.... 79

Chicken Stir-Fry Recipe 82

Vegetable Soup Recipe 84

Breakfast Burrito Recipe 86
Chicken and Vegetable Stir-Fry Recipe 87
Lentil Soup Recipe 89
Stuffed Bell Peppers Recipe 92
Chicken Stir-Fry Recipe 94
Quinoa Salad Recipe 96
Baked Chicken Recipe 98
Chocolate Smoothie Recipe 100
Chicken Salad Recipe 101
Beef Stir-Fry Recipe 103
Lemon Garlic Tilapia 105
Roasted Chicken Breast with Vegetables 106
Quinoa and Vegetable Stir-Fry 108

CONCLUSION AND RECOMMENDATION 112

CHAPTER 1

INTRODUCTION

Potassium is a mineral that is essential for the proper function of the human body. It is classified as an electrolyte because it carries a positive electrical charge in the body and plays a critical role in maintaining fluid balance, nerve function, muscle contractions, and the proper functioning of the heart. Potassium is also involved in the metabolism of carbohydrates and protein, and it helps to regulate blood pressure.

Potassium is naturally found in many foods, including fruits, vegetables, dairy products, and meats. It is also available in supplement form. The recommended daily intake of potassium varies depending on age, gender, and other factors, but in general, adults need about 2,500-3,000 mg of potassium per day. However, some people may need to limit their intake of potassium due to certain health conditions, such as kidney disease or certain medications that can affect potassium levels.

Reason for a low potassium diet

When blood tests show that your potassium level is 5.5 mmol/L or higher, you may be recommended to follow a low-potassium diet. If you are on hemodialysis, your potassium levels should be kept below 6.0 mmol/L. You are in the safe zone if your potassium values are between 3.5 and 5.3 mmol/L.

Remember that not everyone needs to follow a low-potassium diet and that in some cases, a high-potassium diet may be beneficial for overall health. If you have concerns about your potassium levels or need guidance on your diet, it's best to speak with a healthcare provider or a registered dietitian.

There are several reasons why someone might need a low-potassium diet, including:

Kidney disease: People with kidney disease may not be able to properly filter potassium from their blood, leading to high levels of potassium in the body. In these cases, a low-potassium diet may be necessary to prevent complications such as muscle weakness, irregular heartbeat, and even heart failure.

Certain medications: Some medications, such as potassium-sparing diuretics and ACE inhibitors, can increase potassium levels in the body. In these cases, a low-potassium diet may be necessary to avoid potentially dangerous levels of potassium.

Other medical conditions: People with certain medical conditions, such as Addison's disease, may be at increased risk of high potassium levels. In these cases, a low-potassium diet may be recommended to manage symptoms and prevent complications.

Beneficiaries of a low potassium diet

A low-potassium diet may benefit individuals who have certain medical conditions or take certain medications that can affect potassium levels in the body. Some examples include:

Kidney disease: As mentioned earlier, people with kidney disease may need to limit their potassium intake to prevent high levels of potassium in the blood, which can lead to complications.

Chronic kidney disease: People with chronic kidney disease (CKD) may need to follow a low-potassium diet to prevent further damage to their kidneys.

End-stage renal disease: People with end-stage renal disease (ESRD) who require dialysis may need to follow a low-potassium diet to prevent complications during dialysis.

Heart disease: People with heart disease, especially those with heart failure, may need to limit their potassium intake to prevent complications such as irregular heartbeat.

Certain medications: Some medications, such as potassium-sparing diuretics and ACE inhibitors, can increase potassium levels in the body. In these cases, a low-potassium diet may be necessary to avoid potentially dangerous levels of potassium.

CHAPTER 2

OVERVIEW OF LOW POTASSIUM DIET

Potassium is a mineral present in a variety of foods. It maintains the heart beating regularly, aids in fluid balance, and enables nerves and muscles to function properly.

The kidneys are the primary organs in charge of maintaining the proper amount of potassium in the blood. People who take certain medications or have chronic kidney disease must sometimes restrict or increase the amount of potassium in their diet, as directed by their clinician, to maintain their potassium level close to normal. This article discusses how to consume a low-potassium diet, what a normal potassium level is, and how it is measured in the blood. A distinct discussion of other chronic kidney disease treatments is provided.

A reduced potassium diet restricts the consumption of potassium-rich foods. Potassium is a mineral that is necessary for many bodily functions, including fluid balance, regular heart rhythm, and muscle and nerve function. People with certain medical conditions, such as kidney disease, may need to restrict their potassium intake in some instances to avoid complications. A low-potassium diet usually limits the consumption of potassium-rich foods such as fruits, vegetables, dairy products, nuts, and seeds. The aim is to keep potassium levels in the body safe while still meeting the body's nutritional requirements.

Quantity of potassium needed

In general, experts suggest consuming at least 4700 mg of potassium per day. People with mild to severe chronic kidney disease, defined as kidney function (ie, glomerular filtration rate, or "GFR") less than 45 mL/min (normal is 100 to 120 mL/min), should limit their potassium intake to less than 3000 mg per day [2]. Additional restrictions should be imposed based on lab results and the advice of your clinician. A low potassium diet is described as a daily potassium intake of 2000 to 3000 mg.

A certified dietitian or nutritionist can assist you in developing a low-potassium meal plan. The number of portions you require is determined by your height and weight.

The below plan illustrates recommended potassium food consumption per day:

1. Fruit - Consume one to three portions of low-potassium fruit each day.

2. vegetables - Consume two to three servings of low-potassium veggies per day.

3. Dairy and calcium-rich foods - One to two portions per day of low-potassium options

4. Meat and meat alternatives - 3 to 7 meals of low-potassium options per day (approximately 15 percent of calories)

5. Grains - 4 to 7 portions of low-potassium grains per day

Reasons for following a low-potassium diet

When blood tests reveal that the level of potassium in your blood is 5.5 mmol/L or higher, you may be recommended to adhere to a diet that is limited in potassium. If you are undergoing hemodialysis, you need to make it a priority to maintain potassium levels that are lower than 6.0 mmol/L. Your potassium levels are considered to be in the "secure zone" if they fall between 3.5 and 5.3 mmol/L.

There are several reasons why someone might follow a low-potassium diet.

Some of the most common reasons include: Kidney disease: People with kidney disease may need to follow a low-potassium diet because their kidneys are not able to filter excess potassium from the blood, leading to high potassium levels in the body. High potassium levels can cause complications such as muscle weakness, irregular heartbeat, and even heart attack.

Medications: Certain medications, such as potassium-sparing diuretics and angiotensin-converting enzyme (ACE) inhibitors, can cause potassium levels to rise in the body. In these cases, a low-potassium diet may be recommended to prevent complications.

Gastrointestinal issues: People with digestive disorders such as Crohn's disease, ulcerative colitis, or inflammatory bowel disease may be advised to follow a low-potassium diet if they have difficulty absorbing potassium from food or if they experience diarrhea, which can lead to potassium loss.

Hyperkalemia: Hyperkalemia is a condition where there is too much potassium in the blood. In these cases, a low-potassium diet may be prescribed to lower potassium levels in the body.

Pre- or post-surgery: In some cases, a low potassium diet may be recommended before or after surgery to prevent complications, such as irregular heartbeat, during or after the procedure.

Benefits of a low potassium diet

A low-potassium diet may reduce the burden on the kidneys and maintain potassium levels, which is important for individuals with certain chronic conditions. Potassium is a mineral found in many foods and plays many essential roles in the body, including maintaining fluid balance.

These are some of the advantages of a low-potassium diet, which may differ based on the underlying medical condition that necessitates the diet.

Some overall advantages of a low-potassium diet may include:

1. **Lower risk of complications**: Following a reduced potassium diet can help reduce the risk of complications such as irregular heartbeat, muscle weakness, and heart attack in individuals with kidney disease or

other medical conditions that can produce high potassium levels.

2. **Improved blood pressure control:** According to some research, a low-potassium diet may help lower blood pressure in individuals with hypertension, which is a risk factor for heart disease and stroke.

3. **Reduced digestive symptoms:** Following a low potassium diet may help reduce symptoms such as diarrhea and abdominal pain in individuals with digestive disorders such as Crohn's disease or ulcerative colitis.

4. **Medication management:** For people who take medications that can cause high potassium levels, a low-potassium diet can help avoid complications and ensure the medication is working properly.

5. **Individualized nutrition:** A low-potassium diet is frequently tailored to a person's

unique demands and nutritional requirements. This tailored strategy can help ensure that a person gets the nutrients they require while also managing their condition.

CHAPTER 2

FOODS TO AVOID ON A LOW-POTASSIUM DIET

High potassium fruits

It's also worth noting that the serving amount and ripeness of the fruit can have an impact on its potassium content. Smaller and less ripe fruits contain less potassium than larger and completely ripe ones. Consultation with a healthcare expert or registered dietitian can assist in determining how much of these fruits can be eaten safely on a low-potassium diet.

Many of the foods you already consume contain potassium. The foods mentioned below are high in potassium. If you need to increase the quantity of potassium in your diet, make healthy food decisions by adding the following items to your menu.

Many fresh fruits and veggies are rich in potassium:

- Bananas, oranges, melons, honeydew, apricots, and grapefruit (some dried fruits, such as prunes, raisins, and dates, are also high in potassium)
- cooked spinach
- Broccoli cooked
- Potatoes
- Golden potatoes
- Mushrooms
- Peas
- Cucumbers
- Zucchini
- Zucchini
- Greens with leaves
- Juice from potassium-rich fruits is also an excellent option:
- Orange juice

- Tomato juice
- Prunes liquid
- Apricot juice
- Grapefruit juice
- Milk and yogurt, for example, are rich in potassium (low-fat or fat-free is best).

High potassium vegetables

Some vegetables are high in potassium and may need to be limited to a low-potassium diet.

Here are some examples of high-potassium vegetables:

- Potatoes (including sweet potatoes)
- Tomatoes (and tomato products such as tomato sauce and ketchup)
- Spinach
- Brussels sprouts

- Broccoli
- Beets
- Carrots
- Winter squash
- Pumpkin
- Artichokes

High-potassium protein sources

With 332 milligrams per 3-ounce serving, chicken breast has the most, but beef and turkey breast has 315 and 212 milligrams, respectively. If you don't eat meat but enjoy fish, salmon has 326 milligrams of potassium per 3-ounce serving, while canned tuna has 153 milligrams.

It's also worth noting that the serving size and method of preparation can have an impact on the potassium content of these protein sources. Soaking and rinsing canned beans, for example, can help reduce potassium content, whereas grilling or broiling meats can increase potassium content. Consultation with a healthcare professional or registered dietitian can assist in determining how much of these protein sources can be consumed safely on a low-potassium diet.

Some protein sources are high in potassium and should be avoided when following a low-potassium diet.

Here are a few examples of potassium-rich protein sources:

- Lentils and beans (including kidney beans, navy beans, and lentils)
- Products made from soy (including tofu and soy milk)
- Seeds and nuts (including almonds, pistachios, and pumpkin seeds)
- Fish (including salmon and tuna) (including salmon and tuna)

- Poultry (including chicken and turkey) (including chicken and turkey)
- Beef (including ground beef and steak) (including ground beef and steak)
- Pork (including pork chops and pork tenderloin) (including pork chops and pork tenderloin)

CHAPTER 3

FOODS TO INCLUDE IN A LOW-POTASSIUM DIET

Low-Potassium Foods

The list of high-potassium foods may appear to be lengthy, but keep in mind that for every high-potassium food to avoid, there is at least one low-potassium food to enjoy.

The serving size for these potassium-rich foods is 1/2 cup. You don't want to go overboard. A low-potassium food that is consumed in excess becomes a high-potassium food.

Low-potassium fruits:

- Apples (plus apple juice and applesauce) (plus apple juice and applesauce)
- Blackberries

- Blueberries
- Cranberries
- Cocktail of fruits
- Grapes and their juice
- Oranges de mandarin
- Peaches
- Peaches
- Pineapple juice and pineapple
- Plums
- Raspberries
- Strawberries
- Tangerine
- Watermelon
- Vegetables with a low potassium content:
- Alfalfa seeds
- Asparagus (6 raw spears)
- Broccoli (raw or cooked from frozen)
- Cabbage
- Carrots (cooked) (cooked)

- Celery Cauliflower (1 stalk)
- Half an ear of corn (if on the cob)
- Cucumber
- Eggplant
- Wax beans or green beans?
- Kale
- Lettuce
- Mushrooms in white (raw)
- Onion
- Parsley
- Peas (green) (green)
- Peppers
- Water chestnuts Radish
- Watercress
- Squashes and zucchini

Other low-potassium foods:

- Bread (not whole grain)
- Cake (angel or yellow)
- Coffee (8 ounces)

- Cookies (no nuts or chocolate)
- Noodles
- Pies with Pasta (no chocolate or high-potassium fruit)
- Tea with Rice (16 ounces max)

Here's a concept: Potassium levels in certain vegetables can be reduced through a cooking process known as leaching. This goes well with white and sweet potatoes, carrots, beets, winter squash, and rutabagas.

Procedure for leaching

- Fill a pot halfway with warm water.
- Peel and rinse your vegetable in warm water before slicing it into 1/8-inch thick slices.
- Rinse the slices and soak them for 2 hours in the pot. When you pull them

out, rinse them with warm water once more.
- Drain the water from the pot, refill it, and then cook your vegetable.

If you want to leach multiple vegetables at once, soak them in 10 times the amount of water as vegetables. When cooking them, use five times the amount of water that you would for vegetables.

Ask your doctor or nutritionist how to balance high- and low-potassium foods in each meal based on the amount of potassium that's right for you.

CHAPTER 4

A WEEK'S MEAL PLAN FOR A LOW-POTASSIUM DIET

It's important to note that this is just a sample menu plan; specific foods and portions may need to be adjusted based on individual dietary needs and medical conditions. Working with a healthcare professional or registered dietitian to develop a personalized meal plan that meets your specific needs is recommended.

Monday:

Breakfast:

1 scrambled egg
1 slice of whole-grain toast with 1 tablespoon of low-fat margarine
1 small orange
1 cup of low-potassium coffee or tea

Morning Snack:

1 small apple

2 low-potassium graham crackers

Lunch:

2 slices of whole-grain bread with 2 ounces of low-sodium turkey breast and 1 slice of low-fat cheese

1 small green salad with low-potassium vegetables such as lettuce, cucumber, and carrot

1 tablespoon of low-potassium salad dressing

1 small pear

1 cup of low-potassium beverage such as water or apple juice

Afternoon Snack:

1 small banana

1 low-potassium oatmeal cookie

Dinner:

3 ounces of grilled chicken breast

1 small baked sweet potato

1/2 cup of steamed green beans

1 small dinner roll

1 tablespoon of low-potassium margarine

1 small slice of low-potassium apple pie

1 cup of low-potassium beverage such as water or cranberry juice

Before Bed:

1 small serving of low-potassium vanilla pudding

1/4 cup of low-potassium granola

Tuesday:

Breakfast:

1 small serving of low-potassium oatmeal with 1/2 cup of low-potassium milk and 1 tablespoon of honey

1 small banana

1 cup of low-potassium coffee or tea

Morning Snack:

1 small apple

2 low-potassium rice cakes

Lunch:

1 small turkey wrap with low-potassium vegetables such as lettuce and bell peppers

1 small orange

1 cup of low-potassium beverage such as water or grape juice

Afternoon Snack:

1 small peach

1 low-potassium oatmeal bar

Dinner:

3 ounces of baked salmon

1/2 cup of low-potassium quinoa

1/2 cup of steamed asparagus

1 small dinner roll

1 tablespoon of low-potassium margarine

1 small slice of low-potassium lemon cake

1 cup of low-potassium beverage such as water or lemonade

Before Bed:

1 small serving of low-potassium vanilla yogurt

1/4 cup of low-potassium granola

Wednesday:

Breakfast:

1 small serving of low-potassium pancake with 1 tablespoon of low-potassium syrup

1 small tangerine

1 cup of low-potassium coffee or tea

Morning Snack:

1 small pear

2 low-potassium ginger snaps

Lunch:

1 small chicken salad with low-potassium vegetables such as lettuce, cucumber, and carrot

1 small whole-grain pita

1 small banana

1 cup of low-potassium beverage such as water or orange juice

Afternoon Snack:

1 small apple

1 small serving of low-potassium vanilla yogurt

Dinner:

3 ounces of grilled shrimp

1 small serving of low-potassium brown rice

1/2 cup of steamed broccoli

1 small dinner roll

1 tablespoon of low-potassium margarine

Thursday:

Breakfast:

1/2 cup low-potassium oatmeal

1/2 cup low-potassium milk

1/2 cup sliced strawberries

1 slice whole wheat toast with 1 tsp butter

Snack:

1 small apple

1/4 cup unsalted almonds

Lunch:

Grilled chicken breast (3 oz)

1/2 cup cooked white rice

1/2 cup low-potassium green beans

1 small dinner roll

1 tsp butter

Snack:

1 small pear

1/2 cup low-potassium yogurt

Dinner:

Baked pork chop (3 oz)

Friday

Breakfast:

1/2 cup low-potassium cereal

1/2 cup low-potassium milk

1/2 cup sliced peaches

1 slice whole wheat toast with 1 tsp butter

Snack:

1 small banana

1/4 cup unsalted walnuts

Lunch:

Grilled cheese sandwich made with 2 slices of low-potassium bread and 1 slice of low-potassium cheese

1 small orange

1/2 cup low-potassium vegetable soup

Snack:

1 small apple

1/2 cup low-potassium cottage cheese

Dinner:

Baked chicken breast (3 oz)

1/2 cup cooked white rice

1/2 cup steamed broccoli

1 small dinner roll

1 tsp butter

Snack:

1/2 cup low-potassium ice cream

Saturday

Breakfast:

2 egg whites scrambled

1 slice of low-potassium bread toasted

1/4 avocado sliced

1 small orange

Snack:

1/2 cup low-potassium applesauce

2 low-potassium graham crackers

Lunch:

Grilled chicken breast (3 oz)

1/2 cup low-potassium pasta with marinara sauce

1/2 cup steamed green beans

1 small dinner roll

1 tsp butter

Snack:

1/2 cup low-potassium vanilla yogurt

1/4 cup low-potassium granola

Dinner:

Broiled salmon (3 oz)

1/2 cup low-potassium wild rice

1/2 cup cooked carrots

1 small dinner roll

1 tsp butter

Snack:

1 small peach

1/4 cup unsalted almonds

Sunday

Breakfast:
1/2 cup low-potassium oatmeal with 1 tbsp honey

1/2 cup low-potassium milk

1 small apple

1 slice low-potassium toast with 1 tsp butter

Snack:
1/2 cup low-potassium sliced pears

1/4 cup unsalted sunflower seeds

Lunch:
Tuna salad made with 3 oz canned tuna in water, 1/2 cup low-potassium lettuce, 1/2 cup low-potassium tomatoes, and low-potassium salad dressing

1 small orange

1/2 cup low-potassium vegetable soup

Snack:

1 small banana

1/2 cup low-potassium cottage cheese

Dinner:

Grilled pork chop (3 oz)

1/2 cup low-potassium mashed sweet potatoes

1/2 cup steamed asparagus

1 small dinner roll

1 tsp butter

Snack:

1/2 cup low-potassium vanilla ice cream

1/4 cup low-potassium chocolate chips.

CHAPTER 5

TIPS FOR PREPARING LOW-POTASSIUM MEALS

Cooking techniques to reduce potassium levels

Water cooking, pressure cooking, and microwave cooking all reduced potassium levels in all food categories, especially cereals and derivatives, fruits and derivatives, meats and derivatives, legumes, and leafy and cruciferous vegetables.

Before making any major changes to your diet, consult with a healthcare professional or registered dietitian, particularly if you have a medical condition that necessitates a low-potassium diet.

Soaking: Soaking certain high-potassium foods in water for several hours, such as potatoes and legumes, can help decrease their potassium content.

Here are some cooking methods for lowering potassium amounts in food:

1. **Boiling:** Boiling vegetables for at least 10 minutes in a large quantity of water and then discarding the cooking water can help reduce their potassium levels.
2. **Steaming**: Another method for lowering potassium concentration in vegetables is to steam them. It is essential to note, however, that steaming does not remove as much potassium as boiling.
3. **Blanching**: Blanching vegetables in boiling water for a few seconds and then

rinsing them in cold water can help decrease potassium levels.

4. **Grilling and roasting**: By allowing the fat to drip away, grilling and roasting meats can help decrease their potassium content. However, high-potassium marinades and condiments should be avoided.

5. **Using low-potassium ingredients**: Using low-potassium ingredients like low-potassium vegetables, fruits, and grains can help reduce a meal's total potassium content.

Flavorings and seasonings to use

Potassium is found in small quantities in dried mint, oregano, thyme, and sage, ranging from 8 to 19 milligrams per gram. Drinking herbal teas and seasoning meals with these lower-potassium herbs will help you get a little additional potassium.

It is critical to use potassium-free spices and flavorings when following a low-potassium diet. Check the labels of seasonings and flavorings to ensure they are low in potassium, as some mixes may contain high-potassium components such as salt substitutes or dehydrated vegetables.

Here are some alternatives:

1. **Herbs:** Herbs like parsley, thyme, oregano, rosemary, and basil are low in potassium and can contribute flavor to meals.
2. **Spices**: Spices like cinnamon, nutmeg, ginger, and cumin are low in potassium and can be used in both sweet and savory recipes.
3. **Lemon or lime juice:** Lemon and lime juice can add flavor to foods without adding potassium. They can be used in

marinades, vegetable dressings, and sauces.

4. **Vinegar**: Vinegar, such as apple cider vinegar or balsamic vinegar, is low in potassium and can be used in marinades, vegetable dressings, and sauces.

5. **Garlic and onion powder**: Garlic and onion powder are low in potassium and can be used to flavor meats, veggies, and soups.

6. **Mustard**: Mustard is low in potassium and can be used as a condiment or in vegetable dressings.

Tips for eating out on a low-potassium diet

Here are some tips for eating out on a low-potassium diet:

Plan: Before going out to eat, check the menu online to see if there are any low-potassium options available. Many restaurants now have their menus available online.

Speak with the restaurant server: Once you arrive at the restaurant, inform your server about your dietary restrictions and ask if they can provide low-potassium options or modify dishes to make them low-potassium.

Be cautious with sauces and dressings: Many sauces and dressings are high in potassium, so it is important to ask for them on the side or choose low-potassium options such as lemon juice, vinegar, or low-potassium salad dressing.

Choose low-potassium proteins: Lean proteins such as grilled chicken or fish are often low in potassium. Avoid high-potassium proteins such as beef, pork, and organ meats.

Be mindful of sides: Many sides such as mashed potatoes, baked beans, and spinach are high in potassium. Choose low-potassium options such as green beans or a side salad with low-potassium dressing.

Avoid salt substitutes: Salt substitutes often contain potassium chloride, which can be dangerous for those on a low-potassium diet. Stick to regular salt in moderation.

Consider bringing your condiments: If you are unsure if a restaurant's condiments contain potassium, consider bringing your low-potassium options such as lemon juice or low-potassium salad dressing.

Strategies for grocery shopping on a low-potassium diet

Here are some grocery-buying tips for people on a low-potassium diet:

1. Plan your meals: Before you go shopping, plan out your week's meals based on reduced-potassium foods. This will make it simpler to prepare a shopping list and avoid foods high in potassium.

2. Shop the perimeter of the store: Fresh produce, meat, and dairy sections are typically found around the perimeter of most grocery stores. These regions are more likely to have low potassium options.

3. Read food labels: Before purchasing, look for nutrition labels and verify the potassium content of foods. Choose foods with less than 200 mg of potassium per portion.

4. Keep low-potassium staples on board: such as brown rice, whole wheat pasta, low-potassium fruits and veggies, lean proteins such as chicken and fish, and unsweetened almond milk.

5. Avoid high-potassium foods: Bananas, citrus, potatoes, tomatoes, spinach, and avocado are all high in potassium.

6. Consider frozen or canned options: Depending on where you reside, fresh produce may be scarce. Frozen or canned fruits and veggies are acceptable as long as no salt or sugar is added. Check the labels for the potassium level.

7. Speak with a registered dietitian: A registered dietitian can assist you in developing a grocery list and meal plan that fits your particular dietary requirements. They can also teach you how to read food labels and make better food decisions.

CHAPTER 6

RECIPES FOR A LOW-POTASSIUM DIET

Grilled Chicken with Mango Salsa

Ingredients:

4 boneless, skinless chicken breasts

2 ripe diced mangoes,

1 small diced red onion,

1 jalapeño pepper, seeded and diced

1 tbsp lime juice

1 tbsp honey

1/4 tbs salt

1/4 tbs black pepper

Cooking spray

Directions:

Preheat the grill to medium-high.

Combine diced mango, red onion, jalapeo pepper, lime juice, honey, salt, and black pepper in a mixing dish. Place away.

Season the chicken breasts with salt and black pepper after spraying them with cooking spray.

Grill the poultry for 5-6 minutes per side, or until done.

Serve the chicken with the mango sauce on top.

Baked Salmon with Lemon and Dill

Ingredients:

4 salmon fillets

1 tbsp olive oil

1 tbsp fresh dill, chopped

1 sliced lemon

Salt and black pepper, to taste

Directions:

Prepare the oven to 375°F.

Place the salmon fillets in a baking tray.

Drizzle with olive oil and top with parsley.

Season with salt and black pepper.

Place lemon segments on top of each fillet. Bake for 15-20 minutes, or until the salmon is cooked through.

Serve immediately with extra lemon wedges, if desired.

Quinoa Salad with Roasted Vegetables

Ingredients:

1 cup quinoa, rinsed and drained

2 cups low-sodium chicken or vegetable broth

2 cups mixed vegetables (such as zucchini, bell peppers, eggplant, and asparagus), chopped

2 cloves garlic, minced

1 tbsp olive oil

Salt and black pepper, to taste

1/4 cup crumbled feta cheese

1/4 cup chopped fresh parsley

Directions:

Prepare the oven to 400°F.

Toss mixed veggies with garlic and olive oil in a large mixing bowl. Season with salt and black pepper.

Place the veggies on a baking sheet and roast for 20-25 minutes, or until tender and lightly browned.

Meanwhile, cook the quinoa in reduced-sodium chicken or veggie broth according to package directions.

In a big mixing dish, combine the cooked quinoa and roasted vegetables. Top with crumbled feta cheese and minced fresh parsley.

Serve hot or chilled.

Sweet Potato and Black Bean Chili

Ingredients:

1 large sweet potato, peeled and diced

1 can low sodium black beans, drained and rinsed

1 can low-sodium diced tomatoes

1 onion, chopped

2 cloves garlic, minced

1 tbsp olive oil

2 tbsp chili powder

1 tbsp ground cumin

1/4 tbs cayenne pepper

Salt and black pepper, to taste

2 cups low-sodium chicken or vegetable broth

Directions:

Heat the olive oil in a large saucepan over medium heat.

Sauté diced onion and minced garlic for 2-3 minutes, or until onion is translucent.

Add diced sweet potato, black beans, diced tomatoes, chili powder, cumin, cayenne pepper, salt, black pepper, and low-sodium chicken or veggie broth.

Bring to a boil, then lower heat and simmer for 20-25 minutes, or until

Grilled Vegetable Skewers

Ingredients:

1 zucchini, sliced into rounds

1 yellow squash, sliced into rounds

1 red bell pepper, seeded and cut into chunks

1 yellow bell pepper, seeded and cut into chunks

1 red onion, cut into chunks

8 wooden skewers, soaked in water for 30 minutes

2 tbsp olive oil

2 cloves garlic, minced

1 tbsp dried oregano

Salt and black pepper, to taste

Directions:

Preheat the grill to medium-high fire.

Alternate the colors of the veggies on skewers.

In a small dish, combine the olive oil, minced garlic, dried oregano, salt, and black pepper.

Brush the skewered veggies with the olive oil mixture.

Grill for 8-10 minutes, or until veggies are tender and lightly charred, turning periodically.

Serve hot as a side dish or over quinoa or brown rice for a full meal.

Lemon and Herb Baked Chicken

Ingredients:

4 boneless, skinless chicken breasts

2 tbsp olive oil

2 tbsp lemon juice

2 cloves garlic, minced

1 tbsp dried thyme

1 tbsp dried rosemary

Salt and black pepper, to taste

Directions:

Prepare the oven to 375°F.

In a small dish, combine the olive oil, lemon juice, minced garlic, dried thyme, dried rosemary, salt, and black pepper.

Place the chicken breasts in a baking tray.

Brush the chicken breasts with the olive oil mixture, making careful to coat all sides.

Bake for 20-25 minutes, or until the poultry is cooked through and no longer pink in the center.

Take from the oven and set aside for 5 minutes before serving.

Serve with steamed green beans or roasted root veggies for a complete meal.

Quinoa Salad with Roasted Vegetables

Ingredients:

1 cup quinoa, rinsed and drained

2 cups water

1 small eggplant, diced

1 red bell pepper, seeded and diced

1 small zucchini, diced

1 small red onion, diced

2 cloves garlic, minced

2 tbsp olive oil

Salt and black pepper, to taste

1/4 cup chopped fresh parsley

2 tbsp lemon juice

Directions:

Prepare the oven to 400°F.

Toss eggplant, red bell pepper, zucchini, red onion, minced garlic, olive oil, salt, and black pepper in a large mixing dish.

Spread the veggies in a single line on a baking sheet and roast for 20-25 minutes, or until tender and lightly browned.

Meanwhile, bring the quinoa and water to a boil in a medium pot over high heat. Reduce heat to medium, cover, and cook for 15-20 minutes, or until quinoa is tender.

In a large mixing dish, combine cooked quinoa, roasted vegetables, chopped fresh parsley, and lemon juice.

Serve warm or chilled as a side dish or as a light dinner on its own.

Turkey and Vegetable Stir-Fry

Ingredients:

1 pound turkey breast, cut into strips

2 tablespoons olive oil

1 red bell pepper, seeded and sliced

1 yellow bell pepper, seeded and sliced

1 small zucchini, sliced

1 small yellow squash, sliced

1 small onion, sliced

2 cloves garlic, minced

1/4 cup low-sodium chicken broth

2 tbsp soy sauce

1 tbsp honey

1 tbsp cornstarch

Salt and black pepper, to taste

Cooked brown rice, for serving

Directions:

Warm the olive oil in a big skillet or wok over medium-high heat.

Stir-fry the turkey pieces for 3-4 minutes, or until browned and cooked through. Set away after removing from skillet.

Add red bell pepper, yellow bell pepper, zucchini, yellow squash, onion, and minced garlic to the same pan. 3-4 minutes, or until the veggies are tender-crisp.

In a small mixing dish, combine the chicken broth, soy sauce, honey, and cornstarch.

Pour the sauce over the veggies and toss to coat.

Return the cooked meat to the skillet, stirring to combine.

To taste, season with salt and black pepper.

Over prepared brown rice, serve.

Salmon and Asparagus Foil Packets

Ingredients:

4 4-ounce salmon fillets

1 pound asparagus, trimmed

2 tbsp olive oil

1 lemon, thinly sliced

4 cloves garlic, minced

Salt and black pepper, to taste

Directions:

Prepare the oven to 400°F.

Cut four 12x12-inch pieces of aluminum foil. Divide the asparagus evenly among the four squares of foil, arranging it in a single layer in the middle.

Place one salmon fillet on top of each mound of asparagus.

Drizzle olive oil over each fillet, then garnish with lemon segments and minced garlic.

Season with salt and black pepper to flavor. Seal the foil by folding the edges up and over the salmon and asparagus.

Low Potassium Turkey Chili

Ingredients:

1 pound ground turkey

1 can (15 oz) low-sodium black beans, drained and rinsed

1 can (14.5 oz) no salt added diced tomatoes

1 can (6 oz) with no salt added tomato paste

1 onion, chopped

1 green bell pepper, chopped

1 red bell pepper, chopped

2 cloves garlic, minced

1 tbsp chili powder

1 tbsp ground cumin

1/2 tbs smoked paprika

1/4 tbs cayenne pepper

Salt and pepper to taste

1 cup low-sodium chicken broth

Instructions:

In a large pot or Dutch oven, cook the ground turkey over medium-high heat until browned, breaking up any big pieces with a spoon.

Combine the onion, green and red bell peppers, and garlic in a mixing bowl. Cook, stirring periodically until the vegetables are tender.

To the pot, add the chili powder, powdered cumin, smoked paprika, and cayenne pepper. To mix, stir everything together.

To the pot, add the black beans, diced tomatoes, tomato paste, and chicken stock. To mix, stir everything together.

Bring the chili to a boil, then reduce to medium heat. Cook, covered, for 20-30 minutes, stirring periodically.

Season to flavor with salt and pepper. Consume immediately.

Low Potassium Vegetable Stir-Fry

Ingredients:

2 tbsp vegetable oil

1 onion, chopped

1 bell pepper, sliced

2 cloves garlic, minced

2 cups sliced mushrooms

1 cup chopped broccoli

1 cup chopped carrots

1/2 cup chopped celery

1 tbsp low-sodium soy sauce

Salt and pepper to taste

Instructions:

Heat the vegetable oil in a big skillet or wok over medium-high heat.

In the pan, combine the onion, bell pepper, and garlic. Cook, stirring periodically until the vegetables are tender.

In the pan, combine the mushrooms, broccoli, carrots, and celery. Cook, stirring periodically until the vegetables are tender. Drizzle the soy sauce over the veggies, then stir to combine.

Season to flavor with salt and pepper. Consume immediately.

Low Potassium Baked Salmon

Ingredients:

4 salmon fillets

1 lemon, sliced

2 tbsp olive oil

Salt and pepper to taste

Instructions:

Prepare the oven to 375°F.

Place the salmon fillets in a baking tray. Drizzle the olive oil over the fish, then season with salt and pepper.

Top each salmon fillet with a few segments of lemon.

Bake in the preheated oven for 15-20 minutes, or until the salmon is cooked through and flakes readily with a fork.

Serve heated.

Roasted Red Pepper and Feta Salad Recipe

Ingredients:

2 red bell peppers, roasted and sliced

4 oz. crumbled feta cheese

2 cups baby spinach leaves

1/4 cup chopped red onion

1/4 cup chopped fresh parsley

1 tbsp. red wine vinegar

1/4 cup olive oil

Salt and pepper to taste

Instructions:

Prepare the oven to 425 degrees Fahrenheit. Remove the seeds and stems from the red bell peppers and position them cut-side down on a baking sheet. Cook for 20 to 25 minutes, or until the epidermis is blackened and blistered.

Remove the peppers from the oven and put them in a plastic bag or a plastic-wrapped bowl. Allow them to cool for 10-15 minutes before peeling off the skin and slicing them into pieces.

Combine the roasted red peppers, feta cheese, baby spinach leaves, chopped red onion, and fresh parsley in a large mixing dish.

To prepare the dressing, whisk together the red wine vinegar, olive oil, salt, and pepper in a separate small bowl.

Toss the salad with the dressing to coat it equally. Serve directly or refrigerate for later use. Enjoy!

Spicy Grilled Shrimp Skewers Recipe

Ingredients:

1 lb. large shrimp, peeled and deveined

1 tsp. smoked paprika

1 tsp. cumin

1 tsp. garlic powder

1/2 tsp. cayenne pepper

Salt and pepper to taste

2 tbsp. olive oil

Lemon wedges for serving

Instructions:

Preheat the griddle to medium-high.

Combine the smoked paprika, cumin, garlic powder, cayenne pepper, salt, and pepper in a small mixing dish.

Thread the shrimp onto the skewers, leaving room between each prawn.

Brush the shrimp skewers with olive oil, then sprinkle with the spice combination on both sides.

Grill the skewers for 2-3 minutes per side, or until the shrimp are pink and faintly charred.

Remove the skewers from the griddle and drizzle with fresh lemon juice before serving. Enjoy!

Greek Yogurt Chicken Salad Recipe

Ingredients:

2 cups cooked chicken breast, chopped

1/2 cup plain Greek yogurt

1/4 cup chopped celery

1/4 cup chopped red onion

1/4 cup chopped cucumber

2 tbsp. chopped fresh dill

2 tbsp. lemon juice

Salt and pepper to taste

Instructions:

In a large mixing dish, combine the cooked chicken breast, Greek yogurt, celery, red onion, cucumber, and fresh dill.

Stir in the lemon juice, salt, and pepper to flavor.

Refrigerate the bowl for at least 30 minutes to enable the flavors to meld.

Serve the chicken salad on a bed of lettuce, or as a sandwich or tortilla. Enjoy!

Quinoa and Black Bean Salad Recipe

Ingredients:

1 cup cooked quinoa

1 can black beans, drained and rinsed

1/2 red bell pepper, chopped

1/2 yellow bell pepper, chopped

1/4 cup chopped red onion

1/4 cup chopped fresh cilantro

2 tbsp. olive oil

1 tbsp. red wine vinegar

Salt and pepper to taste

Instructions:

Combine the cooked quinoa, black beans, chopped red bell pepper, chopped yellow bell pepper, chopped red onion, and chopped fresh cilantro in a large mixing dish.

Whisk together the olive oil and red wine vinegar in a small dish.

Toss the lettuce with the dressing to coat.

Season with salt and pepper to flavor.

Refrigerate the bowl, covered with plastic wrap, for at least 30 minutes to enable the flavors to meld.

As a side meal or light lunch, serve the salad cold. Enjoy!

Baked Salmon with Lemon and Herbs Recipe

Ingredients:

4 salmon fillets

1 lemon, sliced

1 tbsp. chopped fresh thyme

1 tbsp. chopped fresh rosemary

2 cloves garlic, minced

2 tbsp. olive oil

Salt and pepper to taste

Instructions:

Prepare the oven to 375°F (190°C).

Line a baking dish with aluminum foil and spray with olive oil.

Season the salmon fillets with salt and pepper to flavor.

Top each fillet with lemon segments, chopped fresh thyme, chopped fresh rosemary, and minced garlic.

Drizzle the fish with olive oil.

Bake the salmon for 15-20 minutes, or until the flesh is cooked through and flakes readily with a fork.

Serve the salmon hot, garnished with extra lemon slices and herbs if preferred. Enjoy!

Spicy Shrimp Stir-Fry Recipe

Ingredients:

1 lb. raw shrimp, peeled and deveined

1 red bell pepper, chopped

1 yellow bell pepper, chopped

1 onion, chopped

3 cloves garlic, minced

1 tbsp. fresh ginger, grated

1 tbsp. sesame oil

1 tbsp. low-sodium soy sauce

1 tsp. sriracha sauce

Salt and pepper to taste

Cooked brown rice for serving

Instructions:

Heat the sesame oil in a big skillet or wok over medium-high heat.

Stir-fry the diced onion for 2-3 minutes, or until softened.

Stir in the diced bell peppers, minced garlic, and grated ginger for another 2-3 minutes.

Add the raw shrimp to the pan and stir-fry for 3-4 minutes, or until the shrimp are pink and opaque.

In a small mixing dish, combine the low-sodium soy sauce and sriracha sauce.

Pour the sauce over the shrimp and veggie mixture and toss to coat.

To taste, season with salt and pepper.

Serve the spicy shrimp stir-fry over prepared brown rice. Enjoy!

Quinoa Salad with Roasted Vegetables Recipe

Ingredients:

1 cup quinoa, rinsed and drained

2 cups low-sodium chicken broth or water

1 small eggplant, diced

1 small zucchini, diced

1 red bell pepper, chopped

1 yellow onion, chopped

2 cloves garlic, minced

2 tbsp. olive oil

Salt and pepper to taste

1/4 cup chopped fresh parsley

1/4 cup chopped fresh basil

1/4 cup crumbled feta cheese (optional)

Instructions:

Preheat the oven to 400°F (200°C).

Arrange the diced eggplant, diced zucchini, chopped red bell pepper, and chopped yellow onion on a baking sheet.

Drizzle the vegetables with olive oil and season with salt and pepper to taste.

Roast the vegetables in the oven for 20-25 minutes, until tender and lightly browned.

Meanwhile, bring the low-sodium chicken broth or water to a boil in a medium saucepan.

Add the rinsed and drained quinoa to the saucepan and stir to combine.

Reduce the heat to low, cover the saucepan, and simmer the quinoa for 15-20 minutes, until tender and all of the liquid has been absorbed.

In a large bowl, combine the cooked quinoa and roasted vegetables.

Add the minced garlic, chopped fresh parsley, and chopped fresh basil to the bowl and stir to combine.

If desired, sprinkle the quinoa salad with crumbled feta cheese.

Serve the quinoa salad warm or chilled. Enjoy!

Chicken Stir-Fry Recipe

Ingredients:

2 boneless, skinless chicken breasts, sliced into thin strips

2 cups sliced low-potassium vegetables, such as green beans, carrots, and bell peppers

2 cloves garlic, minced

2 tbsp. low-sodium soy sauce

1 tbsp. rice vinegar

1 tsp. honey

1/4 tsp. red pepper flakes

1 tbsp. vegetable oil

1/4 cup chopped fresh cilantro (optional)

Instructions:

In a small mixing dish, combine the low-sodium soy sauce, rice vinegar, honey, and red pepper flakes. Set away.

In a big skillet or wok over high heat, heat the vegetable oil.

Cook the sliced chicken in the pan for 5-7 minutes, or until browned and cooked through.

Stir-fry the sliced veggies for 3-4 minutes, or until crisp-tender.

Stir in the chopped garlic for 30 seconds, or until fragrant.

Pour the soy sauce mixture over the poultry and vegetables in the skillet.

Cook for 1-2 minutes, stirring constantly until the sauce has thickened and coated the chicken and vegetables.

Remove the skillet from the heat and sprinkle the chicken stir-fry with chopped fresh cilantro, if desired.

Serve the chicken stir-fry over brown rice or with a side of steamed low-potassium vegetables. Enjoy!

Vegetable Soup Recipe

Ingredients:

2 tbsp. olive oil

1 large onion, chopped

2 garlic cloves, minced

2 cups chopped low-potassium vegetables, such as carrots, celery, zucchini, and green beans

4 cups low-sodium chicken or vegetable broth

1 bay leaf

1/4 tsp. dried thyme

1/4 tsp. black pepper

Salt, to taste

1/4 cup chopped fresh parsley (optional)

Instructions:

In a large soup saucepan, heat the olive oil over medium heat.

Sauté the chopped onion in the saucepan for 5-7 minutes, or until soft and translucent.

Sauté the minced garlic in the saucepan for 30 seconds, or until fragrant.

Toss in the chopped low-potassium veggies and stir to combine.

Pour in the low-sodium chicken or veggie broth.

To the saucepan, add the bay leaf, dried thyme, and black pepper.

Bring the soup to a boil, then lower to low heat and continue to cook for 20-25 minutes, or until the vegetables are tender.

Season the soup to flavor with salt.

Take the bay leaf out of the broth.

Ladle the broth into bowls and top with fresh parsley, if preferred.

Serve the veggie soup immediately and enjoy!

Breakfast Burrito Recipe

Ingredients:

2 large eggs

2 tbsp. milk

1/4 cup of low-potassium vegetables, such as diced bell peppers, onions, and spinach

1/4 cup shredded low-potassium cheese

2 small whole wheat tortillas

Salt and pepper, to taste

Salsa, for serving (optional)

Instructions:

In a small dish, whisk together the eggs and milk until well combined.

Heat a nonstick skillet over medium heat and add the low-potassium veggies. Sauté the veggies until tender, about 5-7 minutes. Pour the egg mixture into the pan with the veggies and cook, stirring periodically, until the eggs are set and cooked through about 5-7 minutes.

Sprinkle the grated low-potassium cheese over the eggs and allow it to melt slightly.

Warm the whole wheat tortillas in the microwave for 10-15 seconds, or until they are pliable.

Place the egg and vegetable mixture in the middle of each tortilla.

Roll each sheet into a burrito, tucking in the ends as you go.

Serve the breakfast burritos hot with salsa, if preferred.

Enjoy your reduced potassium breakfast burrito!

Chicken and Vegetable Stir-Fry Recipe

Ingredients:
1 pound boneless, skinless chicken breasts, cut into small cubes
1 tbsp. cornstarch
2 tbsp. vegetable oil

2 cloves garlic, minced

1/2 cup sliced mushrooms

1/2 cup sliced carrots

1/2 cup sliced bell peppers

1/2 cup sliced onions

1/4 cup low-sodium chicken broth

2 tbsp. low-sodium soy sauce

1 tsp. honey

Salt and pepper, to taste

2 cups cooked white rice, for serving

Instructions:

Mix the chicken cubes and cornstarch in a large bowl until the chicken is evenly covered.

In a large pan or wok, heat the vegetable oil over medium-high heat.

Add the chicken to the pan and cook, stirring every so often, for about 5 to 7 minutes, until the chicken is browned and cooked through.

Stir-fry the garlic, mushrooms, carrots, bell peppers, and onions for about 5 to 7 minutes, or until the vegetables are soft.

Whisk the chicken broth, low-sodium soy sauce, and honey together in a small bowl. Pour the sauce over the chicken and vegetables that have been stir-fried and mix everything until the sauce is spread evenly.

Add salt and pepper to taste the stir-fry.

Serve the stir-fried chicken and vegetables over hot white rice.

Enjoy your chicken and vegetable stir-fry that is low in potassium.

Lentil Soup Recipe

Ingredients:

1 tbsp. olive oil

1 onion, chopped

2 cloves garlic, minced

2 carrots, peeled and chopped

2 celery stalks, chopped

1 cup dried green lentils, rinsed and drained

4 cups low-sodium chicken or vegetable broth

1 bay leaf

1/2 tsp. dried thyme

Salt and pepper, to taste

1 tbsp. chopped fresh parsley, for garnish

Instructions:

Heat the olive oil in a large pot over medium-high heat.

Add the onion, garlic, carrots, and celery to the pot and cook, stirring occasionally, until the vegetables are tender about 5-7 minutes.

Add the lentils, low-sodium chicken or vegetable broth, bay leaf, and dried thyme to the pot and stir everything together.

Bring the soup to a simmer and let it cook, uncovered until the lentils are tender about 30-35 minutes.

Remove the bay leaf from the soup and discard it.

Use an immersion blender or transfer the soup to a blender in batches and puree until the soup is smooth and creamy.

Season the soup with salt and pepper, to taste.

Ladle the soup into bowls and garnish each serving with a sprinkle of chopped fresh parsley.

Enjoy your delicious and low-potassium lentil soup!

Stuffed Bell Peppers Recipe

Ingredients:

4 bell peppers, any color

1 lb. ground beef

1/2 cup uncooked white rice

1 onion, diced

2 cloves garlic, minced

1 can (14.5 oz) diced tomatoes, drained

1 tsp. dried oregano

1 tsp. dried basil

Salt and pepper, to taste

1 cup low-sodium chicken or vegetable broth

1/2 cup shredded low-potassium cheese, optional

Chopped fresh parsley, for garnish

Instructions:

Heat the oven to 375°F.

Cut the tops off the bell peppers and remove the seeds and membranes from the inside.

In a big bowl, mix the ground beef, uncooked white rice, diced onion, minced garlic, diced tomatoes, dried oregano, dried basil, salt, and pepper.

Stuff the mixture into the bell peppers, filling them about 3/4 of the way.

Place the stuffed bell peppers in a baking dish and pour low-sodium chicken or vegetable broth over them.

Cover the dish with foil and cook for 45 minutes.

Remove the foil from the dish and, if using, sprinkle the shredded low-potassium cheese on top of the bell peppers.

Return the dish to the oven and bake, uncovered, for another 10 to 15 minutes, or until the cheese is melted and bubbly.

Take the stuffed bell peppers out of the oven and let them rest for a few minutes before serving.

Top each serving with chopped fresh parsley.

Enjoy your tasty and low-potassium stuffed bell peppers!

Chicken Stir-Fry Recipe

Ingredients:

1 lb. boneless, skinless chicken breasts, cut into bite-sized pieces

1/4 cup low-sodium soy sauce

2 tbsp. cornstarch

2 tbsp. water

2 tbsp. vegetable oil

1 red bell pepper, seeded and sliced into thin strips

1 green bell pepper, seeded and sliced into thin strips

1 small onion, sliced

2 cloves garlic, minced

1/2 tsp. ground ginger

Salt and pepper, to taste

Cooked white rice, for serving

Instructions:

In a small mixing dish, combine the low-sodium soy sauce, cornstarch, and water. Place away.

In a big skillet or wok, heat the vegetable oil over medium-high heat.

Stir-fry the chicken chunks in the skillet for 5-7 minutes, or until cooked through.

Stir in the sliced bell peppers and onion for an additional 3-5 minutes, or until the veggies are tender-crisp.

Stir in the minced garlic, ground ginger, salt, and pepper for 1-2 minutes, or until fragrant.

Stir-fry the poultry and vegetables in the skillet for an additional 1-2 minutes, or until the sauce has thickened and coated everything equally.

Remove the chicken stir-fry from the pan and serve over cooked white rice.

Relish your delicious, low-potassium chicken stir-fry!

Quinoa Salad Recipe

Ingredients:

1 cup quinoa, rinsed and drained

2 cups water

1/4 cup chopped fresh parsley

1/4 cup chopped fresh cilantro

1/4 cup chopped fresh mint

1 red bell pepper, seeded and chopped

1 small cucumber, peeled, seeded, and chopped

1 small red onion, chopped

1/4 cup fresh lemon juice

2 tbsp. olive oil

Salt and pepper, to taste

Instructions:

In a medium saucepan, mix the rinsed quinoa and water. Bring to a boil over a high fire.

Reduce the heat to medium, cover the saucepan, and cook for 15-20 minutes, or until the quinoa is tender and the water has been absorbed.

Remove the saucepan from the flame and set aside to cool to room temperature.

In a large mixing dish, combine the cooked quinoa, fresh parsley, cilantro, mint, red bell pepper, cucumber, and red onion.

In a small mixing dish, combine the fresh lemon juice and olive oil. Season with salt and pepper to flavor.

Toss the quinoa salad with the lemon juice and olive oil dressing in a big mixing bowl until everything is well combined.

Refrigerate the quinoa salad for at least 30 minutes, or until cold before serving.

Enjoy your delectable, low-potassium quinoa salad!

Baked Chicken Recipe

Ingredients:

4 boneless, skinless chicken breasts

1/4 cup low-sodium chicken broth

2 tbsp. olive oil

1 tsp. dried thyme

1 tsp. dried oregano

1/2 tsp. garlic powder

Salt and pepper, to taste

Instructions:

Preheat your oven to 375°F.

In a small bowl, whisk together the low-sodium chicken broth, olive oil, dried thyme, dried oregano, garlic powder, and salt and pepper to taste.

Place the boneless, skinless chicken breasts in a baking dish.

Pour the chicken broth and olive oil mixture over the chicken breasts, making sure they are coated evenly.

Bake the chicken in the preheated oven for 20-25 minutes or until the internal temperature of the chicken reaches 165°F.

Remove the baking dish from the oven and let the chicken rest for a few minutes before slicing and serving.

This low-potassium baked chicken recipe is easy to prepare and makes a delicious and healthy main dish for your low-potassium diet!

Chocolate Smoothie Recipe

Ingredients:

1/2 cup unsweetened almond milk

1/2 banana, frozen

1 tbsp. unsweetened cocoa powder

1 tbsp. almond butter

1/2 tsp. vanilla extract

1-2 ice cubes

Instructions:

In a blender, combine the unsweetened almond milk, frozen banana, unsweetened cocoa powder, almond butter, vanilla extract, and 1-2 ice pieces.

Blend on high until smooth and buttery.

If the smoothie is too thick, add a little more almond milk until the desired consistency is achieved.

Pour the smoothie into a tumbler and serve.

This low-potassium chocolate smoothie recipe is a delicious way to satiate your sweet appetite without exceeding your daily potassium limit. It's also high in protein and healthy fats, so you'll feel full and satiated.

Chicken Salad Recipe

Ingredients:

2 cups cooked chicken breast, chopped

1/2 cup celery, diced

1/2 cup red onion, diced

1/4 cup plain Greek yogurt

1/4 cup mayonnaise

1 tbsp. Dijon mustard

1 tbsp. lemon juice

Salt and pepper to taste

Instructions:

Mix the chopped poultry, celery, and red onion in a large mixing bowl.

Whisk together the Greek yogurt, mayonnaise, Dijon mustard, and lemon juice in a second small mixing bowl until well combined.

Toss the poultry mixture in the dressing until evenly coated.

To taste, season with salt and pepper.

Serve the chicken salad over greens or with low-potassium crackers or bread.

This low-potassium chicken salad recipe is a delicious and simple lunch or dinner choice. The tangy taste and creaminess of the Greek yogurt and Dijon mustard are enhanced without adding too much potassium. Furthermore, the chicken contains enough protein to keep you full and content.

Beef Stir-Fry Recipe

Ingredients:

1 lb. beef sirloin, thinly sliced

1 red bell pepper, sliced

1 green bell pepper, sliced

1 small onion, sliced

2 cloves garlic, minced

1 tbsp. vegetable oil

1 tbsp. low-sodium soy sauce

1 tbsp. cornstarch

1/4 cup beef broth

Salt and pepper to taste

Instructions:

In a small mixing bowl, whisk together the soy sauce, cornstarch, and beef broth. Set aside.

Heat the vegetable oil in a large skillet over high heat.

Add the beef and cook until browned on all sides, about 5-7 minutes.

Add the bell peppers, onion, and garlic to the skillet and stir-fry for an additional 3-4 minutes, or until the vegetables are crisp-tender.

Pour the soy sauce mixture over the beef and vegetables and stir until everything is well coated.

Reduce the heat to medium and cook for an additional 2-3 minutes, or until the sauce has thickened and the beef is cooked through.

Season with salt and pepper to taste.

Serve the beef stir-fry over a bed of low-potassium rice or noodles.

This low-potassium beef stir-fry recipe is a delicious and nutritious meal that's easy to make at home. The beef provides a good source of protein, while the bell peppers and onion add vitamins and fiber. Plus, the low-sodium soy sauce and cornstarch help to keep the potassium levels in check. Enjoy this dish as a flavorful and filling dinner option.

Lemon Garlic Tilapia

Ingredients:

4 tilapia fillets

2 cloves garlic, minced

2 tablespoons lemon juice

1 tablespoon olive oil

1 teaspoon dried basil

Salt and pepper, to taste

Instructions:

Preheat oven to 400°F (200°C).

Fillets of tilapia should be put in a baking dish.

Mix the garlic, lemon juice, olive oil, basil, salt, and pepper in a small bowl.

Pour the mixture on top of the fillets of tilapia.

Bake for 10-15 minutes or until the fish is cooked through.

Serve hot with the sides you choose.

Note: You can easily change this recipe to include the vegetables and starches of your choice, as long as they are low in potassium.

Roasted Chicken Breast with Vegetables

Ingredients:

4 boneless, skinless chicken breasts

2 cups chopped mixed vegetables (e.g. carrots, zucchini, bell peppers, onions)

2 tablespoons olive oil

2 cloves garlic, minced

1 teaspoon dried thyme

Salt and pepper, to taste

Instructions:

Preheat oven to 400°F (200°C).

Line a baking sheet with parchment paper.

Arrange the chicken breasts on the baking sheet and season with salt, pepper, and thyme.

In a large bowl, mix the chopped vegetables, olive oil, garlic, salt, and pepper.

Spread the vegetable mixture around the chicken on the baking sheet.

Roast for 25-30 minutes or until the chicken is cooked through and the vegetables are tender.

Serve hot with your choice of low-potassium starches.

Note: You can use any combination of low-potassium vegetables in this recipe. Just make sure they are chopped to a similar size for even cooking.

Quinoa and Vegetable Stir-Fry

Ingredients:

1 cup uncooked quinoa

2 cups low-sodium chicken or vegetable broth

2 tablespoons vegetable oil

2 cloves garlic, minced

2 cups mixed vegetables (e.g. bell peppers, broccoli, carrots, onions)

1 tablespoon low-sodium soy sauce

1 tablespoon rice vinegar

1 teaspoon sesame oil

Salt and pepper, to taste

Instructions:

Rinse the quinoa under running water in a fine-mesh strainer.

Bring the quinoa and stock to a boil in a medium saucepan over high heat.

Reduce the heat to medium, cover, and cook for 15-20 minutes, or until the quinoa is tender and the liquid has been absorbed.

Heat the vegetable oil in a big skillet or wok over high heat.

Cook for 1 minute, or until the garlic is aromatic.

Stir-fry the mixed veggies for 5-7 minutes, or until tender-crisp.

Combine the prepared quinoa, soy sauce, rice vinegar, sesame oil, salt, and pepper in a mixing bowl.

Cook for another 2-3 minutes, or until everything is thoroughly heated.

As a reduced potassium main course, serve hot.

In this recipe, you can use any mix of low-potassium vegetables. Just make certain they Rinse the quinoa under running water in a fine-mesh strainer.

Bring the quinoa and stock to a boil in a medium saucepan over high heat.

Reduce the heat to medium, cover, and cook for 15-20 minutes, or until the quinoa is tender and the liquid has been absorbed.

Heat the vegetable oil in a big skillet or wok over high heat.

Cook for 1 minute, or until the garlic is aromatic.

Stir-fry the mixed veggies for 5-7 minutes, or until tender-crisp.

Combine the prepared quinoa, soy sauce, rice vinegar, sesame oil, salt, and pepper in a mixing bowl.

Cook for another 2-3 minutes, or until everything is thoroughly heated.

As a reduced potassium main course, serve hot.

In this recipe, you can use any mix of low-potassium vegetables.

CHAPTER 7

CONCLUSION AND RECOMMENDATION

It is important to consult with a healthcare provider if you have concerns about your potassium levels or are considering making significant changes to your diet. You should consult with a healthcare provider

if you have kidney disease, heart disease, or other conditions that affect potassium levels, are taking medications that affect potassium levels, are experiencing symptoms of high or low potassium levels, are pregnant or breastfeeding, or have questions about your diet or nutrition.

Your healthcare provider or a registered dietitian can provide guidance and advice to ensure that you're getting the appropriate amount of potassium for your individual needs.

People with kidney problems or other health conditions that require them to restrict their potassium intake should follow the standard advice and eat a low-potassium diet. Potassium is a mineral that is necessary for the body to sustain fluid and electrolyte balance. However, both too much and too little potassium can create a variety of health issues.

Bananas, tomatoes, avocados, potatoes, spinach, and a wide variety of other fruits, vegetables, and cereals are rich in potassium. Meals low in potassium, on the other hand, include most meats, bread, grains, and certain fruits and vegetables such as pears, blueberries, and green beans.

If you are on a low-potassium diet, you must work closely with your healthcare practitioner or a registered dietitian to ensure that you are getting enough potassium to meet your specific requirements. They may counsel you to include or avoid certain foods, as well as give you recipes for potassium-rich meals. They may also offer guidance on food preparation.

Recommendations for sticking to a potassium-deficient diet:

Following a potassium-deficient diet can be difficult, but here are some useful hints:

1. Create a personalized meal plan with the assistance of a healthcare practitioner or a certified dietitian that meets your nutritional needs while also lowering your potassium intake.

2. Pay close attention to the labels and ingredient lists on packaged foods to

identify potassium-rich foods and avoid consuming them. Consider keeping a food diary to track how much potassium you consume regularly.

3. Choose foods with reduced potassium content, such as white rice, spaghetti, bread, sugar-free cereals, and canned or frozen fruits and veggies.

4. Remember the proper portion sizes. Even foods with minimal potassium content can quickly add up if consumed in excess.

5. Try experimenting with various herbs and seasonings instead of using high-potassium ingredients like salt, soy sauce, or tomato sauce to flavor your food.

6. Consider various cooking methods that have the potential to help lower the potassium content of specific foods, such as boiling potatoes or vegetables in a large

amount of water and then draining the water after cooking.

While on a low-potassium diet, make sure to take any medications prescribed to you precisely as directed, and notify your healthcare provider if you notice any new or worsening symptoms.

Made in United States
North Haven, CT
14 June 2024